What Plan Is

BEST FOR YOU
As a
WEIGHT WATCHER

Dr. Benjamin O Williams

Table Of Contents

INTRODUCTION

Might it be said that you are a veggie lover, vegetarian, Entire Food Plant Based, or just eating fewer creature items while following the WW focuses framework? Peruse on to figure out how to find lasting success with the WW plan for weight reduction utilizing the Weight Watchers Individual Focuses plan.

MODULE ONE: What's The Best Weight Watchers Plan for Vegetarians?

The Weight Watchers (WW) framework is perfect for weight reduction for veggie lovers and vegetarians.
Weight Watchers Individual Focuses on Veggie lovers and Vegans
In November of 2021, WW presented the new Private Focuses plan that offers every part an extraordinary food evaluation test and fosters your customized day-to-day focused remittance and zero-point food list.

Since the Individual Focuses plan is customized to your necessities, you can make the WW program function admirably for you to eat a veggie-lover, vegetarian, or entire food, plant-based way of life despite everything getting more fit.

Remember the accompanying tips.

- Pick beans and tofu as your protein sources
- Pick entire grains you appreciate like oats, potatoes, or corn.
- If you eat eggs, pick eggs as an extra protein source.
- Pick avocado as a solid fat on the off chance that that is a food you appreciate and eat routinely.
- If you eat organic products routinely, click yes during the test and it will be no focus for you.

The choices you pick during the test will turn into your zero-point food varieties, which is an incredible advantage as a WW veggie lover since you will not need to count focuses for these sound, filling food sources.

If you will quite often utilize more pre-arranged vegan food sources (like veggie burgers, frozen feasts, oils, spreads, and vegetarian cheeses, you might need to take the appraisal and pick less protein and sugar decisions. This will give you all the more everyday focus.

On the off chance that you are diabetic, the test will naturally relegate focus to you for sugar food sources, including organic products. This is a piece trickier to explore as a veggie lover or vegetarian however should in any case be possible effectively.

My more seasoned WW Plan - What's the Best WW Variety Plan for Veggie Lovers?

Note: The My WW Plan with Green, Blue, and Purple is presently not accessible. If you have any desire to follow a past WW anticipate your own, you can utilize this My WW Purple aide or utilize the application track nibbles which have comparable forms to past Weight Watchers plans.

The WW purple arrangement is best for veggie lovers, vegetarians, and those following a plant-based, meatless way of life.

Here's the reason the Weight Watchers (WW) purple arrangement is best for vegans:

- You don't need to focus on all leafy foods. These most quality food varieties are not focused on WW Purple and ought to be most of your eating regimen.
- You don't need to count the focus for entire grains. Entire grains have focuses on different plants, they are not focused on purple which leads you normally to

pick oats, earthy colored rice, and other filling starches.

- You don't need to count focus for beans. Beans are magnificently solid, filling food that is ideally suited for dropping pounds. Since they are not focused on WW, you can eat beans, lentils, tofu, and edamame to get all the filling protein and sustenance you want.
- You don't need to count focuses for potatoes. Indeed, potatoes are a weight reduction food! Here is an extraordinary rundown of sound potato recipes that are low in focus.
- You don't need to focus on bland vegetables. Food sources like corn, popcorn, oak seed squash, and butternut squash can be a customary piece of your eating regimen without the need to follow them.

Since your everyday focus recompense is lower, you will not be enticed to gorge on vegetarian low-quality foods or an excessive amount of solid fat. Quite possibly the main motivation why veggie lovers and vegans are overweight is because they depend on vegetarian low-quality foods like handled veggie burgers, vegetarian cheddar, and vegetarian chips, saltines, and treats. These food sources have focused on WW Purple and this is something to be thankful for. Solid fats like coconut oil and nuts have focus as well so you will not indulge them.

- Prepared potatoes in a bowl

Potatoes are delectable, filling weight reduction food and they are not focused on WW purple.

10 Tips for Vegetarians and Vegans on Weight Watchers Green, Blue, and Purple Plans

Here are the best tips for vegetarians and vegans on WW:

1. Limit or dispense with high-fat dairy assuming you are vegan. Some of the time individuals change to a vegan diet and tragically load up on dairy all things considered. (Requesting the cheddar enchiladas rather than the chicken ones, for instance.) This isn't helping your body, particularly with weight reduction.
2. Limit or dispose of veggie lover low-quality food. There's a spot in this world

for vegetarian substitution food varieties like veggie burgers, vegetarian cheddar, and nibble food varieties. Yet, it should be a tiny, once-in-for a little while treating part of your eating regimen. The WW focuses framework will assist you with this because handled food varieties have focus and genuine food sources are practically every one of the zero places. Indeed, Oreos are vegetarian yet they aren't assisting you with shedding pounds.

3. Eat genuine food. A big part of every plate I eat is vegetables. I eat those first. The other half is solid starches like entire grains, potatoes, and beans. I eat essentially, the food is delectable, I'm seldom eager, and it's exceptionally low in calories.

4. Load up on vegetables. You turned into a veggie lover which is as it should be. You need to eat plants! Vegetables are your companion. Eat a gigantic assortment of them consistently. Here is an extraordinary rundown of ways of eating more vegetables.

5. Lessen or dispose of the oil. Oil has been promoted for a long time as solid. the food however is astute advertising, not

reality. Either cut back or dispose of oils from your eating regimen, even coconut, and olive oil. Here is an extraordinary rundown of sans oil salad dressings to utilize.

6. Limit solid fats. I used to nibble on modest bunches of nuts, generously add avocado to everything, and eat peanut butter off the spoon a few times each day when I went into the storage space. Indeed, our bodies need fat, however just a tiny sum.

7. Abstain from gorging. An excessive amount of food is a lot of food, regardless of how solid it is.

8. Pick entire grains and potatoes (tacky starches) over dry ones. Cooked earthy colored rice, potatoes, and entire wheat pasta are superbly filling and nutritious. There are likewise no focuses on WW purple. Pretzels and chips are vacant calories and won't keep you full.

9. Track your focus. This is valid for each WW part and it's valid for vegans. You joined Weight Watchers for an explanation, so track your focus. I track every day and I wouldn't have it differently.

10. Feast prep one time each week. Planning food is significant for every individual who needs to get more fit yet this is particularly evident on the off chance that you follow a plant-based way of life. Spend an hour or so toward the end of the week making a bunch of rice, cooking a solid bean soup or stew, and hacking a few vegetables and natural products. You'll be headed to a breathtaking week.

***NOTE:** Chocolate banana frozen yogurt in a bowl Banana pleasant cream is a great WW vegan bite or sweet - it poses a flavor like delicate frozen yogurt.*

My Green, Blue, and Purple Plans Made Sense

The Weight Watchers framework recently had 3 variety plans for individuals to look over. The program has now changed to the Weight Watchers Customized Focuses Plan as of November 2021.

- Weight Watchers Green Arrangement - Individuals get 100 zero-point food sources (products of the soil) and somewhere around 30 every day focuses.

- Weight Watchers Blue Arrangement - Individuals get 200 zero-point food varieties (organic products, vegetables, lean proteins) and no less than 23 everyday places.

- Weight Watchers Purple Arrangement - Individuals get 300 zero-point food varieties (natural products, vegetables, proteins, entire grains, and potatoes) and something like 16 every day every day

Which Weight Watchers plan is the most famous? The vast majority follow the WW Blue arrangement.

The most effective method to Pick the MyWW Program for You

When a weight reduction of 130 pounds. Change to an Entire Food, consider a Plant-Based way of life to mend stomach-related issues and as of now utilize the WW Purple arrangement. I love it!

When you're at your objective weight, change to a plant-based diet and hope to get in shape, however, lose 25 extra pounds and joyfully be in the center of my weight territory.

Do Weight Watchers Work for Veggie Lovers and Vegetarians?

Indeed, WW is a well-conceived plan for getting thinner with a plant-based way of life.

Weight reduction is about calories. (WW utilizes focus to assist you with dealing with your calories.) It doesn't make any difference if you are following a low carb, high carb, vegetarian, keto, or some other kind of diet. Weight reduction possibly happens when you eat fewer calories than you consume, and the WW focuses framework will show you how to do that.

MODULE TWO: Best Recipes For Weight Watchers

1 . Weight Watchers Hotcakes

Quite possibly the best thing about Weight Watchers is that it's not prohibitive.

Not at all like a few different eating regimens where you cut out entire nutrition types, WW permits everything from tacos to pizza.

Try to design. Thus, assuming that you realize you're having pizza for supper, perhaps decide on something with fewer focus for lunch.

In any case, if you realize supper is a sound chicken serving of mixed greens, you can without much of a stretch enjoy a part of these yummy hotcakes.

Also, remember, that most organic products are inconsequential, so you can top these with a wide range of berries.

2. Weight Watchers Apple Oats Biscuits

Biscuits are a dynamite method for beginning your day, yet they're not very 'diet' cordial.

Fortunately, this Weight Watchers recipe will top you off and fulfill your sweet tooth without utilizing all your day-to-day focuses.

Stacked with genuine apples, oats, and earthy-colored sugar, this preference is more like a thick oats treat. There's additionally a lot of warmth from the cinnamon.

3. Weight brunchZero Point Cabbage Soup

The excellence of picking Weight Watchers is that you can gobble up every one of the organic products on and veggies you like, and it doesn't combine with your day-to-day places.

I don't look at, however, any eating regimen that advises me to remove berries, bananas, and new veggies don't sound that compelling to me.

Be that as it may, for this situation, the rundown of zero-point food varieties is longer than a CVS receipt.

So go ahead and top this soup up with any extra vegetables you could have in the ice chest.

4. Weight Watchers Pizza

Can we just be real for a minute — pizza is what we miss the most while we're attempting to practice good eating habits, correct?

With the delicate, delicate base and the lashings of sauce and cheddar on top, I wind up dreaming about it.

I don't believe there's a more ideal food than pizza!

This extraordinary two-fixing batter is similar to the one used to make thin bagels. All you'll require is Greek yogurt and self-rising flour.

To attempt this before focusing on a major pack of flour you probably won't utilize once more, take a stab at making your own.

Simply add 1 1/2 teaspoons of baking powder and 1/4 teaspoon of salt to one cup of regular flour.

5. Weight Watchers Parmesan Chicken Cutlets

Crunchy chicken generally involved digging it in flour and egg followed by a mix of breadcrumbs and Parmesan cheddar.

I like to butterfly chicken bosoms so they cook quicker, however, go ahead and keep them entire assuming that you like them.

One way or another, you shouldn't have any issues keeping the covering set up with no eggs. Simply don't deal with the chicken a lot after it's plunged.

6. Weight Watchers French Bread Rolls Recipe

Following quite a while of being told carbs are the foe, specialists are currently saying that cutting carbs can adversely influence your well-being.

Carbs and gluten are not awful for you as we've been made to accept. All things being equal, very much like some other nutrition class, you want to direct the amount you eat.

So kindly, eat the bread! It's flavorful, delicate, and wonderful with a smear of salted spread. Also, at only four places, it merits consistency.

Weight Watchers Chicken Serving of mixed greens with Grapes
My Insane Great Life
This Weight Watchers Chicken Serving of mixed greens is tasty and thus simple to get ready! I love involving rotisserie chicken for this, as it is an efficient recipe! Serve this on lettuce, make a chicken plate of mixed greens, or use it in a sound chicken plate of mixed greens sandwich-it depends on you!

7. Weight Watchers Chicken Serving of mixed greens with Grapes

I love a chicken serving of mixed greens, and I'll cheerfully eat it in a bowl all alone.

Ordinarily, I'll make it with bacon pieces, mayo, and perhaps slashed bubbled eggs for added protein.

This recipe has a shrewd stunt to eliminate those calories.

As opposed to adding mayo, you'll add without fat plain yogurt and olive oil mayo for a magnificently velvety and similarly rich completion.

The grapes, apples, and nuts will give you a lot of surfaces and exquisite pleasantness, and you can add bubbled eggs, as well, on the off chance that you need them.

8. Rosemary Cooked Potatoes Recipe

French fries probably won't be the most ideal decision while you're watching your weight, however broiled potatoes are incredible as a side dish.

They're delicate, fresh on the edges, and being heated, they're solid. To such an extent that they're on the zero-point records.

These likewise incorporate olive oil, garlic, rosemary, and salt and pepper, so this is certainly not a zero-point dish.

9. Weight Watchers Zucchini Corn Squanders Recipe

Corn squanders are radiant, sweet, and fresh, and work out positively for everything from salmon to cooked pork.

These additionally incorporate zucchini for an additional kick of zero-point goodness.

Stary by whisking the eggs with liquefied spread and milk, and make sure to utilize skimmed milk to eliminate the calories.

To that, you'll add the dry blend followed by corn, cheddar, and zucchini.

To hold the zucchini back from making it excessively wet, take a stab at sprinkling some salt over the top and passing on it in a sifter to deplete.

Then, softly press it with a paper towel.

10. Weight Watchers Hamburger and Broccoli

As I would like to think, takeout generally tastes so great since another person made it. It's shrewd, modest, languid, and exactly what you'll require in the wake of a difficult week.

Yet, regardless of whether you're attempting to watch calories on Weight watchers, you can in any case enjoy.

Meat and broccoli are really solid, all things considered, and since this isn't covered in a thick layer and afterward broiled, you can have an additional spoonful.

11. Weight Watchers Cooked Red Pepper Fish Salad

This fish salad is solid, filling, and meets up in under ten minutes.

Simply mix sans fat mayonnaise with non-fat acrid cream and dill until overall quite smooth.

Then, at that point, mix through some diced onion, broiled red peppers, and water-stuffed fish.

I hate dill, so I settled on thyme and scallions all things considered. Likewise, this would work with plain, non-fat yogurt, as well.

12. Weight Watchers Pasta with Garlic Sauce

Legitimate Italian pasta doesn't depend on thick, weighty sauces to make its feasts splendid and delectable.

You're bound to see a major bowl of pasta or spaghetti with just olive oil and garlic than a velvety Alfredo sauce.

Tenderly intensity some olive oil and mix in the parsley and garlic. Keep it moving until it's fragrant, and afterward throw in the pasta.

Polish it off the intensity with a liberal measure of Parmesan cheddar on top.

13. Slow Cooker Break Chicken

Between the cream cheddar, bacon, and cheddar, break chicken isn't the best feast on this rundown.

In any case, this recipe calls for without fat cream cheddar and dry Farm preparing. That scales back such countless calories while as yet making this smooth and delightful.

Furthermore, you'll utilize boneless chicken bosoms, which are loaded with protein and very lean.

14. Weight Watchers Stew

Stew is one of my go-to dinners when I want something simple, filling, and loaded with protein. All you'll require is ground meat, beans, and a couple of key flavors.

Despite the fact that hamburger is more extravagant in flavor, you can undoubtedly utilize something less fatty, similar to chicken or turkey, since you don't taste the meat to such an extent as the flavors and veggies.

That, yet you can mass bean stew out with a wide range of zero-point vegetables as well. I like to add squash or yam alongside corn and even cauliflower.

15. Weight Watchers Chicken Quesadillas

One thing many health improvement plans share practically speaking is their appearing contempt of cheddar.

What's more, Let's get real here for a minute, that is one thing I can't surrender.

So the way that you can besides the fact that cheddar on Weight have Watchers yet that you can have an entire chicken quesadilla for just five focuses is a serious addition to.

Simply make sure to purchase low or diminished fat cheddar. Or on the other hand, in the event that you could do without low-fat cheddar, have a go at utilizing mozzarella with a sprinkle of healthful yeast all things being equal.

16. Weight Watchers Simmered Vegetables - 0 Focuses

In the event that you're searching for a side dish for one of the recipes above yet don't have any desire to squander a lot of your day to day focuses on fries or weighty pasta, this zero-point dish takes care of you.

With the new WW framework, you'll be given a variety plan, and each plan considers somewhat various focuses and fixings.

Thus, check what veggies are no focuses for your arrangement, and afterward broil them with cooking shower, thyme, salt, and pepper.

17. Weight Watchers Szechuan Shrimp Recipe

In addition to the fact that this is just three focuses per segment, however it utilizes storeroom staples and meets up in less than 20 minutes.

Dissimilar to some other Asian-style sauces that require rice vinegar or mirin, all you'll have to make this sauce is ketchup, soy sauce, honey, ginger, red pepper drops, garlic, and green onions.

Serve it with this three-point simple broiled rice from Weight Watchers.

18. Weight Watcher's Corn Chowder

It In the event that you really hate mollusk chowder but rather have a desire for something warm and rich, you need to attempt this corn chowder recipe.

Begin by mellowing the onions and carrots in a Dutch broiler and afterward make a roux with flour, garlic, and veggie stock.

Where different recipes utilize weighty cream, this lower-calorie rendition has you rush a portion of the corn and potato soup to give it a rich and velvety completion.

19. Weight Watchers Fudge Brownies

Weight Watchers and brownies? Might it at some point be valid?

Not exclusively are these chocolatey and heavenly, however they're just 2-3 focuses per segment! With that low number, you might have two.

To keep these low in focuses, you'll utilize almond milk, unsweetened fruit purée sauce, unsweetened cocoa powder, and sugar.

This last fixing assists with keeping these low in calories.

Lakanto Baking Sugar is very much looked into, however evaluate a couple of choices to find the one you like the best.

20. Weight Watchers Apple Fresh

Apple fresh is now really sound when you contrast it with cakes, treats, and brownies.

It's stacked with organic product, and the fixing commonly has oats for added fiber.

Since this has much less sugar than normal apple fresh, I recommend utilizing sweet apples, similar to Fuji or Honeycrisp, as the more delectable apples will stand apart more without the additional sugar.

The other significant replacement in this is the utilization of light spread or margarine. Since this doesn't have to rise, it doesn't require full-fat margarine.

It's simply to assist with restricting the garnish fixings, so you might utilize coconut oil in the event that you needed to, making this vegetarian boot.

21. Pineapple Pastry

This fleecy pineapple cake Is only five/six-point and brimming with astounding fruity flavors.

It's so light, because of the whipped egg whites, which add a lot of air to the hitter. Furthermore, once more, you'll utilize light spread to eliminate calories.

As it's loaded with squashed pineapple, it needn't bother with any icing or whipped cream on top.

22. WW Pan fried Rice

I love broiled rice, yet I think we as a whole know it's not the most solid of feasts.

Obviously, utilizing earthy colored rice, chicken bosom, and low so low-sodium will assist with that.

One more sharp method for keeping this low in focuses is to just utilize the whites of the eggs, which are high in protein however much better for you.

To make this extra sound, utilizing cauliflower rice would trickle the focuses significantly further.

23. 2-Fixing Strawberry Cushion Pastry

Think about what number of WW focuses this sweet little treat has? ZERO! Could you at any point trust it?

We as a whole realize that I have a really heavy sweet tooth, so removing treat isn't a possibility for me. With this delicicus recipe, I can have dessert consistently.

All you'll require is 0% Greek yogurt and without sugar Crystallize O in anything flavor you like.

To get that vaporous, mousse-like surface, whisk the yogurt for 5 minutes, and afterward whisk it with the arranged Solidify O for an additional 10 minutes.

24. Peanut Butter and Banana Short-term Oats

Assuming that your everyday stipend is around 27-29 focuses, chances are, you won't have any desire to 'squander' 15 focuses on a lavish breakfast.

All things considered, it's ideal to adhere to around 1/4 of your day to day focuses with the goal that you have sufficient left over for a generous lunch and supper.

Fortunately, this short-term oat recipe is only five focuses, so you might have a latte close by on the off chance that you need.

The enchanted fixing in this is their peanut butter, which has all the flavor and none of the fat.